SIMPLE SIBO DIET COOKBOOK

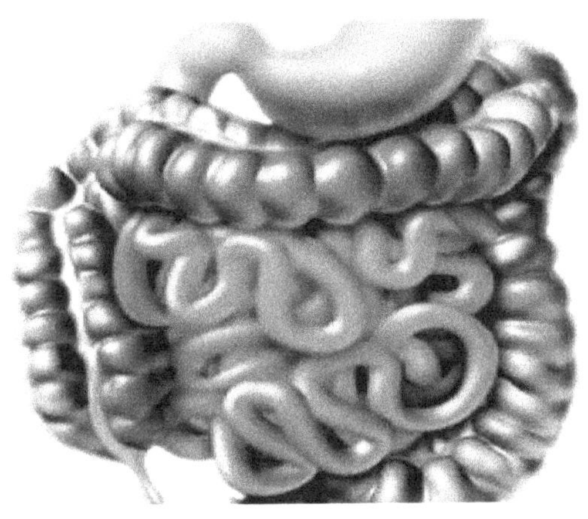

Recipes to Rebalance Health, Relieve Symptoms and Heal Your Gut for Good

Dr Stephanie C. McCarthy

Table of Contents

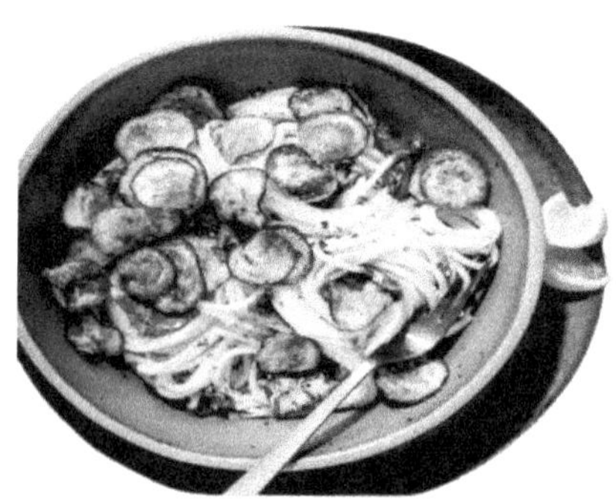

Introduction

John was a retired farmer who lived in a small town with his loving wife, Mary. They had been married for over 50 years, and they were inseparable.

John had always been a healthy man, but in recent years, he had started to feel tired and bloated. He had also lost weight, and he was no longer able to enjoy his favorite foods.

John went to the doctor, who diagnosed him with SIBO, or small intestinal bacterial overgrowth.

The doctor told John that there was no cure for SIBO, but that he could manage it with diet and medication. John was determined to get better, so he started reading everything he could about SIBO.

One day, John's wife, Mary, was doing research about the disease. That's when she came across an article of mine that I wrote about SIBO Disease with recipes that can help rebalance SIBO disease. And how I was able to successfully use the diet to help my patients with SIBO.

Mary decided to start cooking John meals from the recipes. John was skeptical at first, but he was willing to try anything to feel better.

Within a few weeks, John started to feel better. His bloating went away, and he had more energy. He was also able to start eating his favorite foods again.

John continued to follow the SIBO Diet, and after a few months, he was feeling completely healthy. He was so grateful to Mary for finding the diet, and he was determined to share it with others who were struggling with SIBO.

John and Mary's story is a reminder that SIBO is a manageable condition. With the right diet and medication, people can live healthy and fulfilling lives. Their story triggered me to write this book about SIBO Disease, Diet and Meal Plan to help manage SIBO, with the help of this book everyone will be able to rebalance their body and live in health.

One day, John and Mary threw a party to celebrate John's recovery. Their family and friends were all there, and they were all so happy to see John healthy and happy again.

John gave a speech at the party, thanking his wife for her love and support, and thanking the doctors and researchers who had helped him to get better.

He also talked SIBO Diet, and how it had helped him to regain his health.

John's story is an inspiration to anyone who is struggling with SIBO. It shows that it is possible to manage this condition and live a healthy and fulfilling life.

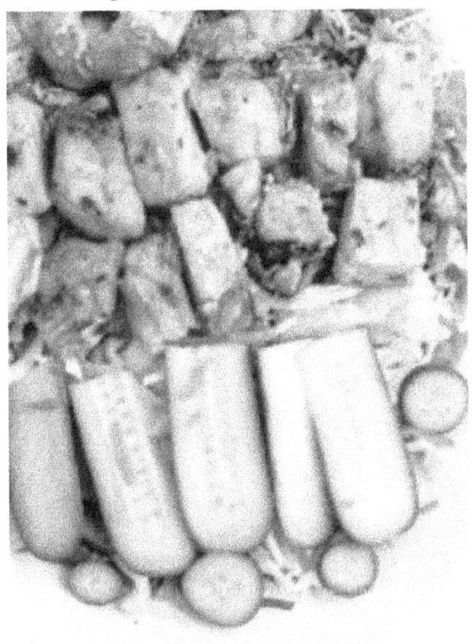

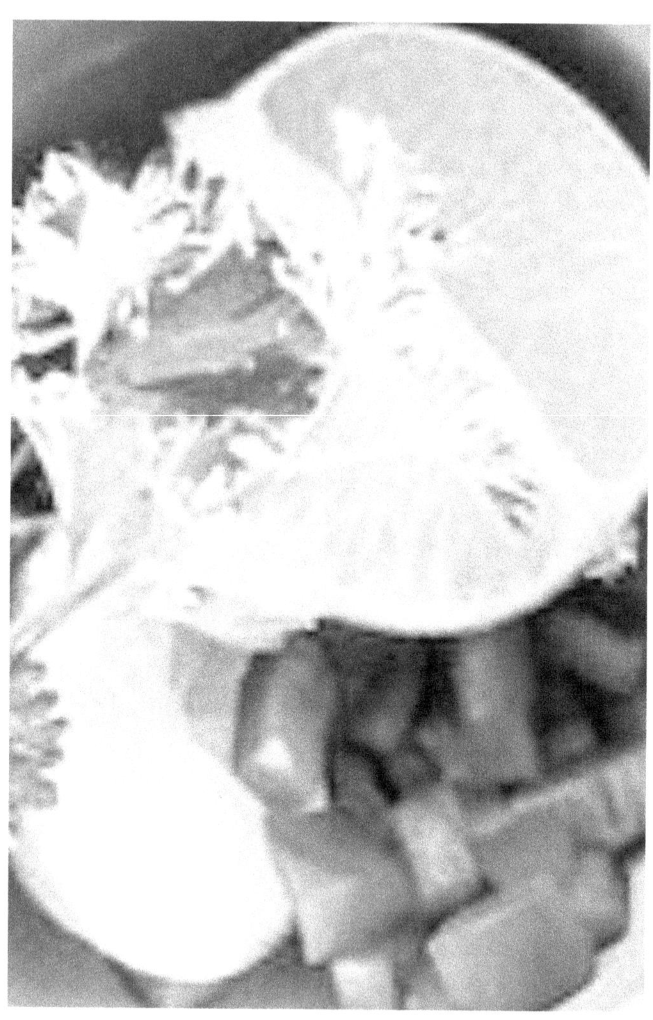

Chapter 1

Small Intestinal Bacterial Overgrowth (SIBO) Demystified:

Types, Causes, Symptoms, and Prevention Measures

Small intestinal bacterial overgrowth, commonly known as SIBO, is a complex digestive disease that affects the small intestine.

This condition occurs when an abnormal number of bacteria (normally found in the colon) colonize the small intestine.

Bacterial overgrowth can interfere with the normal digestive process, causing a range of unpleasant symptoms and potential health complications.

In this book, we'll delve into the complexities of SIBO, including its types, causes, symptoms, and prevention.

Understanding SIBO

The small intestine is necessary for the digestion and storage of nutrients from food. In a healthy digestive tract, the small intestine has a relatively low bacterial population. However, in situations of SIBO, an excessive amount of bacteria from the colon flows towards the small intestine, affecting the nutrient absorption and causing a variety of gastrointestinal symptoms.

Types of SIBO

SIBO is typically classified into two primary types:

1. **Hydrogen-Predominant SIBO (H2-SIBO):** This kind of SIBO can be described as an overgrowth of hydrogen-producing bacteria. When these bacteria ferment undigested carbs, they generate hydrogen gas, which can be detected through breath testing.

2.   **Methane-Predominant SIBO (CH4-SIBO):** In this type, methane-producing bacteria proliferate in the small intestine. Methane gas is produced during the fermentation of carbohydrates, leading to distinct digestive symptoms.

Causes of SIBO

The exact causes of SIBO can be multifaceted and may include:

- **Impaired Motility:** Factors that alter the digestive tract's typical muscular contractions, such as irritable bowel syndrome (IBS) or scleroderma, can impede food transit through the small intestine, allowing germs to collect.

- **Anatomical Abnormalities:** Structural issues like intestinal strictures or diverticula can create pockets where bacteria can thrive.

-**Medications:** Some medications, particularly those that affect stomach acid production or motility, can contribute to SIBO.

- **Underlying Gastrointestinal Conditions:** Conditions such as Crohn's disease or celiac disease can disrupt the balance of gut bacteria and predispose individuals to SIBO.

- Prior Gastrointestinal Surgery:

Surgeries that alter the normal anatomy of the digestive tract can increase the risk of SIBO.

Common Symptoms of SIBO

SIBO can manifest in a variety of symptoms, and their severity may vary from person to person. Common symptoms include:

- **Discomfort in the Abdomen:** SIBO patients frequently report significant stomach pain, bloating, and cramps.

- **Gas and Bloating:** Excess gas is created as a result of bacteria fermenting carbohydrates, resulting in obvious bloating and frequent gas.

- **Constipation or Diarrhea:** SIBO can cause bowel motions to become irregular, resulting in either frequent diarrhea or constipation.

- **Nutritional Shortages:** Bacterial overgrowth can limit the absorption of essential nutrients such as vitamins and minerals, leading in malnutrition over time.

- **Fatigue:** Consistent weariness might result from a combination of stomach discomfort and nutrient loss.

- **Loss of Weight:** SIBO can cause unintentional weight loss, especially when nutrient absorption is significantly hindered.

- **Joint Pain and Skin Conditions:** SIBO can cause systemic inflammation, which can cause joint discomfort and skin problems in some people.

Prevention Measures for SIBO

Preventing SIBO often involves addressing underlying causes and maintaining a diet that minimizes bacterial overgrowth. Here are key preventive measures:

1. Identify and treat any underlying conditions: Work with your healthcare practitioner to handle any illnesses that predispose you to SIBO, such as IBS or Crohn's disease.

2. **Proper Hygiene:** Good hygiene practices, such as frequent handwashing, can help lower the risk of bacterial infection.

3. Avoid unwanted antibiotics: Antibiotics have the potential to disturb the balance of gut microorganisms. Use them only as directed by a healthcare expert.

4. **Balanced Diet:** To reduce bacterial fermentation in the small intestine, have a balanced diet low in fermentable carbohydrates (FODMAPs).

5. **Probiotics: ** Probiotics may be beneficial in some circumstances to reestablish a healthy balance of gut flora; however, before beginning any supplements, contact with a healthcare expert.

6. **Stress Reduction:** Stress can impair intestinal motility and worsen SIBO symptoms.

Stress-reduction practices such as yoga, meditation, or deep breathing exercises should be used.

7. **Regular Check-Ins:** If you have a history of SIBO or are at risk, see your doctor on a frequent basis to monitor your gut health.

Small Intestinal Bacterial Overgrowth (SIBO) is a complicated digestive condition marked by bacterial overgrowth in the small intestine. It can cause a variety of unpleasant symptoms as well as nutritional inadequacies. Understanding the kinds, causes, symptoms, and prevention methods for SIBO is critical for people who are at risk and those who want to properly manage this condition. Individuals can take proactive actions to limit the risk of SIBO and its accompanying symptoms by treating underlying causes and keeping a balanced diet.

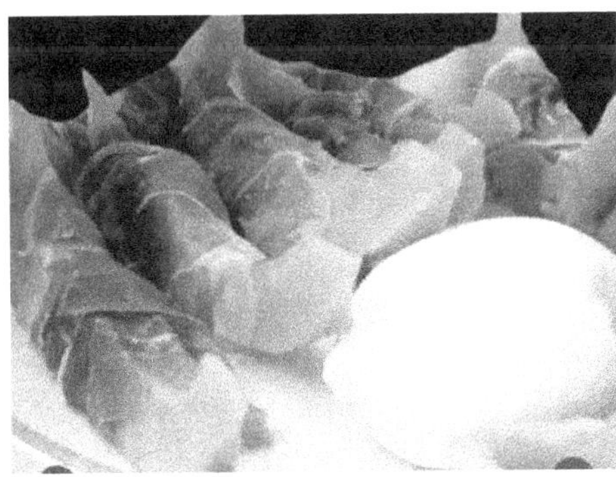

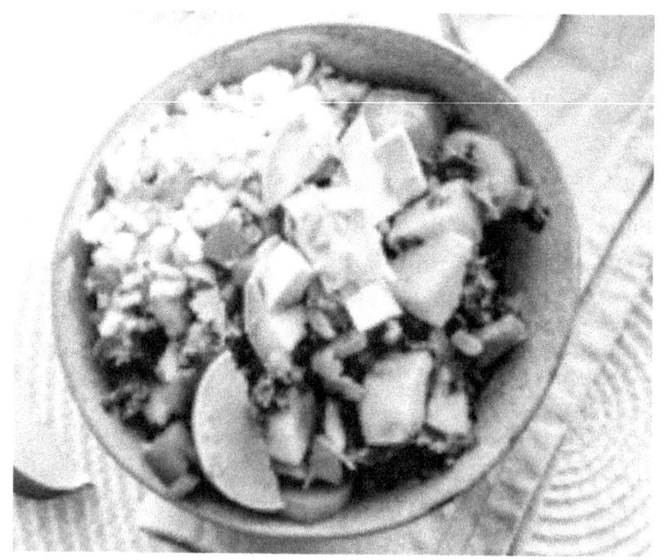

Chapter 2

Foods to Embrace and Avoid for Optimal Health

The Simple SIBO Diet Cookbook provides advise on which foods to include and which to avoid in order to attain optimal health and relieve symptoms. Individuals trying to reclaim control of their gut health must first understand the concepts of a SIBO-friendly diet.

Foods to Embrace

1. **Low-FODMAP Vegetables:** Fermentable oligosaccharides, disaccharides, monosaccharides, and polyols (FODMAPs) are commonly tolerated in vegetables. Spinach, zucchini, carrots, and cucumbers are among examples.

2. **Lean Proteins**: Incorporate lean protein sources such as poultry, fish, and tofu into your diet. These are easy to digest and supply vital amino acids.

3. **Fruits with Low Fructose Content:** Choose low-fructose fruits such as berries, kiwi, and citrus fruits. These have a lower likelihood of exacerbating SIBO symptoms.

4. **Gluten-Free Grains** Many people with SIBO find comfort from gluten-free grains such rice, quinoa, and oats. These grains are less likely to irritate the digestive tract.

5. **Herbs and spices**: Use herbs with antimicrobial qualities, such as oregano, thyme, and rosemary, to help reduce bacterial overgrowth. Ginger and turmeric can help with digestion and inflammation.

6. **Fats:** Healthy fats like olive oil, avocado, and coconut oil are high in nutrients and tolerated well by most SIBO patients.

7. **Bone Broth**: Homemade bone broth is easy on the stomach and rich in minerals. It can be used as a base for soups and stews.

8. **Foods High in Probiotics** Fermented foods such as kefir, yogurt (if tolerated), sauerkraut, and kimchi can help restore a healthy gut flora balance.

9. **Homemade Soups & Broths:** Soups cooked with low-FODMAP veggies, lean meats, and bone broth are nourishing and soothing to the digestive system.

10. **Nutritional Supplements:** If deficiencies are a concern, contact with a healthcare physician before taking certain nutritional supplements such as vitamin B12 or iron.

Foods to Avoid

1. **FODMAP-Rich Foods** Avoid high-FODMAP foods such as garlic, onions, wheat, and certain legumes, since they might aggravate SIBO symptoms.

2. **Sugars and Sweeteners**: Sugar, high-fructose corn syrup, and artificial sweeteners should be avoided since they may feed bacteria and increase overgrowth. If tolerated, use natural sweeteners such as stevia or tiny quantities of maple syrup or honey.

3. **Dairy:** Lactose intolerance is common in SIBO patients. Avoid dairy products or substitute

lactose-free alternatives such as almond milk or lactose-free yogurt.

4. **Grains Containing Gluten:** Wheat, barley, and rye are rich in gluten and may cause SIBO symptoms. Choose gluten-free choices.

5. **Manufactured Foods:** Highly processed meals often include chemicals, preservatives, and artificial components that might irritate the digestive tract. When possible, choose entire, unprocessed meals.

6. **Carbonated Drinks:** Carbonated beverages may cause bloating and discomfort by introducing extra gas into the digestive tract.

7. Caffeine and alcohol: Caffeine and alcohol may both impaired gastrointestinal function and should be eaten in moderation or avoided entirely.

8. **Spicy Foods:** Spicy meals might cause stomach irritation. Limit or avoid them, particularly if they aggravate symptoms.

9. **Fruit Juices:** Fruit juices contain high levels of fructose and may be harmful. Whole fruits are preferable.

10. **Large Meals: ** Large meals might be difficult for the digestive system. Reduce the strain on your digestive system by eating smaller, more frequent meals.

It's crucial to remember that the severity of SIBO symptoms and dietary tolerances might differ across people. Some people may be able to gradually reintroduce specific foods, but others may need to follow a more limited diet.

The SIBO Diet Cookbook presents a set of dietary recommendations emphasizing the necessity of eating foods that are gentle on the digestive system while avoiding those that might aggravate symptoms. Individuals with SIBO may strive toward optimum gut health and increased overall well-being by carefully choosing meals and eating mindfully.

Core Benefits of Following a SIBO Diet Cookbook

Following a SIBO Diet Cookbook provides numerous key advantages for those suffering from Small Intestinal Bacterial Overgrowth (SIBO). These advantages revolve on symptom relief, gut health improvement, and general well-being. Here is a summary of the main advantages, along with explanations:

1. **Relief of Symptoms:** Symptom alleviation is one of the key advantages of following a SIBO Diet Cookbook. Individuals may lessen discomfort and enhance their quality of life by eating foods that are less likely to aggravate SIBO-related symptoms such as bloating, stomach pain, and diarrhea.

2. **Control of Bacterial Overgrowth:** The cookbook focuses on meals that prevent bacterial overgrowth in the small intestine. Individuals may help control and manage SIBO more successfully by avoiding high-FODMAP meals and carbohydrates that feed harmful bacteria.

3. **Improved Digestion:** A SIBO-friendly diet emphasizes readily digested, gentle-on-the-digestive-system foods. This may

result in better digestion, less gas, and less pressure on the stomach.

4. **Nutritional Absorption:** SIBO may interfere with nutritional absorption, resulting in deficits. Individuals may improve their nutritional balance and general health by eating nutrient-dense, readily absorbed meals.

5. **Reduced Inflammation:** Certain items in the SIBO Diet Cookbook, such as anti-inflammatory herbs and spices, may help lower gut inflammation, alleviating inflammation-related symptoms and promoting long-term gut health.

6. **Balanced Gut Microbiome:** Consuming probiotic-rich foods such as yogurt and kefir may aid in the restoration of a healthy balance of gut bacteria. A healthy microbiome is essential for optimal digestion and general health

7. **Adaptable Approach:** The SIBO Diet Cookbook allows you flexibility and personalization. Individuals may tailor their diet to their unique tolerances, preferences, and sensitivities while following the diet's main principles.

8. **Weight Control:** Because of malabsorption, many people with SIBO lose weight unintentionally. A SIBO-friendly diet may help you lose weight by optimizing your nutritional intake and controlling your symptoms.

9. **Increased Energy Levels:** Better digestion and nutrition absorption might contribute to an increase in energy levels. This enables people to participate in everyday tasks with more vigor and less weariness.

10. **Long-Term Gut Health**: A SIBO Diet Cookbook not only treats symptoms but also promotes long-term gut health. Individuals may lower the chance of SIBO recurrence and maintain a healthy digestive tract by adopting long-term eating habits.

11. **Holistic Well-Being**: Managing SIBO with food benefits not just physical health but also mental and emotional well-being. Relieving unpleasant symptoms may help to decrease stress and enhance overall quality of life.

12. **Resource for Education:** The cookbook is an instructional resource, including information about SIBO, nutritional suggestions, and recipes. It

provides people with the information they need to make informed health decisions.

A SIBO Diet Cookbook, in short, provides a holistic approach to controlling the illness by concentrating on symptom treatment, gut health improvement, and general well-being. Individuals may recover control of their digestive health, ease pain, and move toward a better, more balanced life by carefully choosing meals.

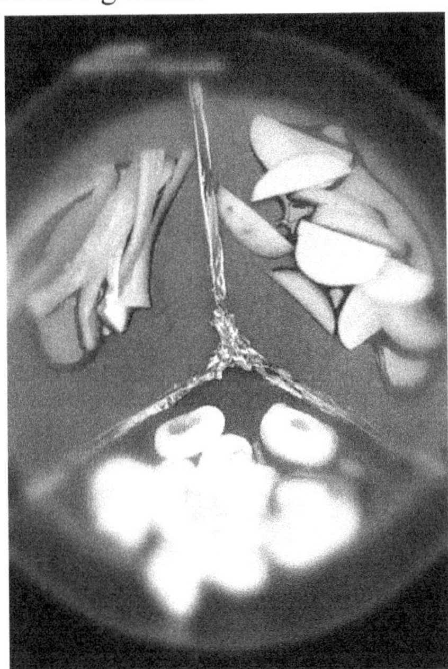

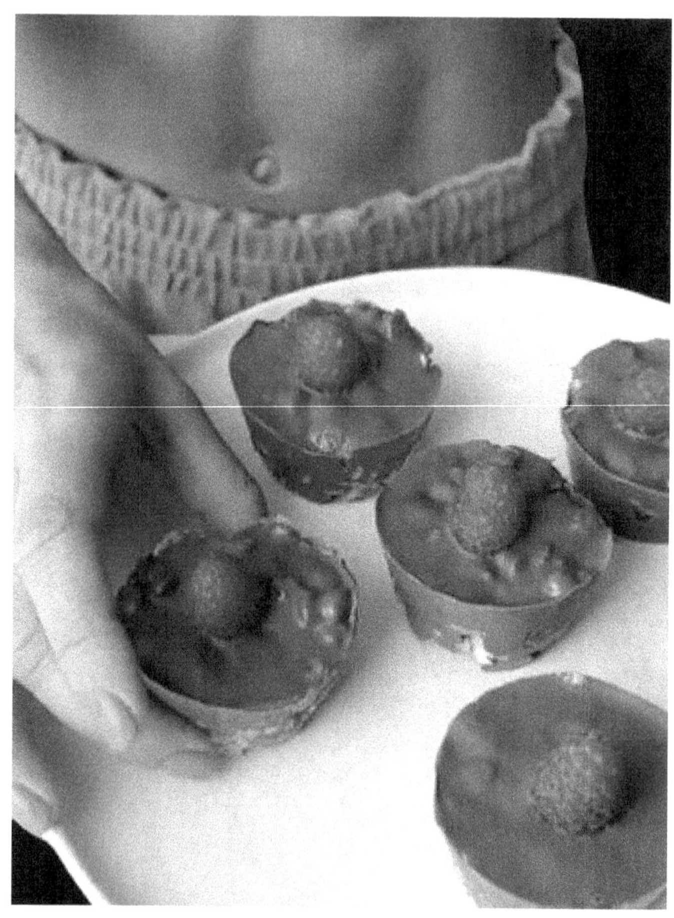

Chapter 3

How to Follow a SIBO Diet Cookbook

Following a SIBO Diet Cookbook entails taking a methodical approach to treating Small Intestinal Bacterial Overgrowth (SIBO) by carefully choosing foods and meals that are less likely to aggravate symptoms. Here's a step-by-step method to successfully implementing a SIBO Diet Cookbook:

1. Understand SIBO Dietary Guidelines: Become acquainted with the SIBO-specific dietary concepts. These usually include limiting or eliminating particular foods that might cause symptoms.

2. Learn to Recognize Safe and Dangerous Foods: - Examine the listings of safe and harmful foods in the cookbook. Foods that are safe are less likely to encourage bacterial overgrowth or to produce symptoms. Unsafe foods should be avoided since they have the potential to aggravate SIBO.

3. Meal Preparation: Plan your meals around SIBO-friendly dishes from the guidebook. Concentrate on choosing meals that adhere to the dietary standards.

4. Grocery Shopping: Make a list of the products you'll need for your SIBO-friendly dishes. Prioritize fresh, natural meals above processed or pre-packaged goods.

5. Cooking Techniques: Become acquainted with cooking methods that increase taste without increasing SIBO symptoms. Gentle sautéing, roasting, and the use of anti-inflammatory herbs and spices are examples of these approaches.

6. Portion Control: Watch your portion amounts. Smaller, more frequent meals might be gentler on the digestive tract and aid with symptom management.

7. Experiment and modify: Experiment with various recipes and modify them to your preferences and dietary restrictions. You may often change the ingredients or spices in recipes to make them more appetizing while still following SIBO guidelines.

8. Maintain a Food journal: - Keep a food journal to chronicle your meals, symptoms, and probable food triggers. This may aid in the identification of certain foods that may be harmful for you.

9. Stay Hydrated: To maintain good digestion, drink plenty of water. Herbal teas and caffeine-free drinks are often well accepted.

10. Monitor Symptoms: Keep track of your SIBO symptoms and make note of any changes. This information may be beneficial to both your healthcare professional and your own knowledge of how your body reacts to certain meals.

11. Gradual Reintroduction (With Supervision): whether your symptoms improve and you're under the supervision of a medical practitioner, you might try gradually reintroducing particular foods to see whether you can tolerate them. This should be done meticulously and methodically.

Patience, dedication, and self-awareness are required while following a SIBO Diet Cookbook. Working closely with healthcare specialists who can provide direction and monitor your development is critical. You may successfully treat SIBO and enhance your overall gut health by following the dietary concepts indicated in the cookbook and making smart food choices.

Healthy Shopping List for a SIBO Diet

When following a SIBO diet, it's critical to pick items that are less likely to aggravate symptoms while still supporting gut health. Here is a list of 20 SIBO-friendly shopping ingredients

1. Lean Proteins:
  - Chicken breast
  - Turkey
  - Lean cuts of beef
  - Fish (e.g., salmon, trout)
  - Tofu or tempeh (if tolerated)

2. Low-FODMAP Vegetables:
  - Spinach
  - Zucchini
  - Carrots
  - Bell peppers
  - Cucumbers

3. Low-Fructose Fruits:
  - Blueberries

   - Strawberries
   - Kiwi
   - Cantaloupe
   - Citrus fruits (e.g., oranges, grapefruits)

4. Gluten-Free Grains:
   - Rice (white or brown)
   - Quinoa
   - Oats (certified gluten-free)
   - Millet

5. Cooking Oils:
   - Olive oil
   - Coconut oil
   - Avocado oil

6. Fresh Herbs and Spices:
   - Oregano
   - Thyme
   - Rosemary
   - Basil
   - Turmeric

7. Low-Lactose Dairy Alternatives:
   - Lactose-free yogurt (if tolerated)
   - Almond milk
   - Coconut milk

8. Homemade Bone Broth:

- Chicken, beef, or vegetable-based bone broths can serve as a base for soups and stews.

9. Eggs:
   - Eggs are typically well-tolerated and versatile for various recipes.

10.   Low-FODMAP   Sweeteners   (in moderation):
   - Stevia
   - Maple syrup (in small amounts)
   - Honey (in small amounts)

11. Nut and Seed Butters (in moderation):
   - Almond butter
   - Sunflower seed butter
   - Peanut butter (if tolerated)

12. Fresh Seafood:
   - Opt for fresh, unprocessed seafood like shrimp, scallops, and mussels.

13.   Low-FODMAP   Legumes   (in moderation):
   - Lentils (small portions)
   - Canned chickpeas (drained and rinsed)
   - Green beans

14. Vinegars (in moderation):

- Rice vinegar
- Apple cider vinegar

15. Nutritional Yeast:
- A flavorful, dairy-free option for adding a cheesy taste to dishes.

16. Fresh Ginger:
- Fresh ginger can aid digestion and add flavor to recipes.

17. Homemade Sauces and Dressings:
- Make your own dressings and sauces using SIBO-friendly ingredients like olive oil, vinegar, and fresh herbs.

18. Low-FODMAP Nuts (in moderation):
- Almonds
- Walnuts
- Pecans (small portions)

19. Probiotic-Rich Foods:
- Fermented foods like lactose-free kefir, sauerkraut, or kimchi (if tolerated).

20. Fresh, Filtered Water:
- Staying hydrated with clean, filtered water is crucial for gut health.

It's important to note that individual tolerances can vary, so it's essential to monitor your body's response to these ingredients and make adjustments accordingly.

SIBO disease complications, if the proper diet is not followed

Small Intestinal Bacterial Overgrowth (SIBO) may lead to a variety of issues and have a detrimental influence on one's health if the proper diet is not followed. Here are some of the possible consequences of untreated or poorly controlled SIBO:

1. **Nutritional Shortages:** SIBO may impair the absorption of vital nutrients such as vitamins (B12, D) and minerals (iron, calcium). This may lead to dietary shortages, anemia, bone health difficulties, and other health problems over time.

2. **Malabsorption:** Malnutrition may result from persistent nutritional malabsorption, which can appear as unexpected weight loss, weakness, exhaustion, and a compromised immune system.

3. **Persistent Gastrointestinal Symptoms:** SIBO-related symptoms such as bloating, stomach

discomfort, diarrhea, or constipation may develop chronic and have a negative influence on a person's quality of life if not treated dietarily.

4. IBD (Inflammatory Bowel Disease): According to some study, there may be a relationship between SIBO and the development or worsening of inflammatory bowel illnesses such as Crohn's disease or ulcerative colitis.

5. **Autoimmune Diseases:** Chronic inflammation in the gut, which is often linked with SIBO, may lead to the development or worsening of autoimmune disorders.

6. **Increased Infection Risk:** SIBO may impair the immune system's function in the stomach, rendering people more vulnerable to gastrointestinal infections.

7. **Intestinal Permeability (Leaky Gut):** SIBO-related inflammation may increase intestinal permeability, often known as "leaky gut." This disorder may enable dangerous compounds to enter the circulation via the gut lining, possibly provoking immunological responses and systemic health consequences.

**8. **Sepsis: ** Untreated SIBO may develop to sepsis, a potentially fatal illness characterized by a systemic infection that can damage numerous organs, in extreme instances.

9. **Minor Intestinal Damage: Chronic SIBO may damage the lining of the small intestine over time, affecting its function and worsening malabsorption concerns.

10. **Increased Risk of SIBO return: Individuals who have successfully treated SIBO may be at risk of return, necessitating further rounds of therapy if dietary and lifestyle modifications are not made.

It is important to note that SIBO is a treatable illness, and by following the appropriate diet, many people receive considerable symptom alleviation and better gut health. Early intervention and a well-managed food plan may assist to avoid these issues and promote overall health.

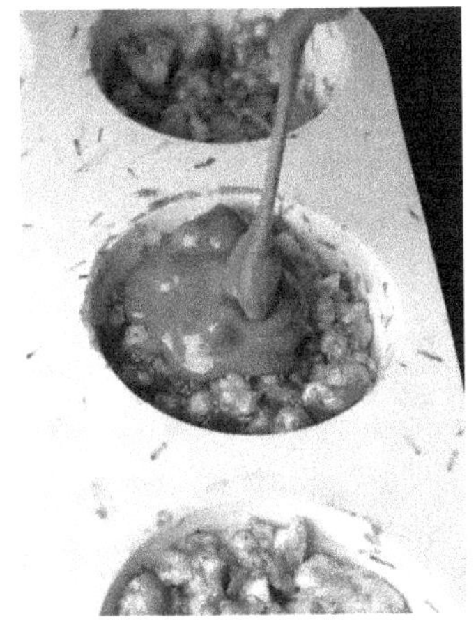

Chapter 4

Meal Planning for SIBO Diet:

Meal planning is an essential part of properly managing a Small Intestinal Bacterial Overgrowth (SIBO) diet. It entails carefully choosing meals, quantity amounts, and mealtimes to reduce discomfort and promote gut health. Here's a description of SIBO diet meal planning and its benefits:

1. Choosing SIBO-Friendly Foods: Meal preparation begins with selecting meals low in fermentable carbohydrates (FODMAPs), sugars, and other elements that might aggravate SIBO symptoms. Lean proteins, low-FODMAP veggies, gluten-free cereals, and particular fruits are examples.

2. Macronutrient Balancing: Aim for macronutrient balance in your meals. To ensure you obtain a mix of nutrients, include lean protein, healthy fats, and carbs (ideally low-FODMAP grains and veggies) in each meal.

3. ****Portion Control****: To prevent overloading your digestive system, watch your meal amounts. Smaller, more frequent meals may be simpler to digest and may aid with symptom management.

4. ****Home Cooked Meals:**** Making your own meals provides you control over the ingredients and enables you to tailor recipes to your dietary requirements. It is simpler to avoid hidden FODMAPs and sugars in handmade foods.

Benefits of Meal Planning for SIBO Management:

1. **Symptom Management:** Meal planning guarantees that you eat SIBO-friendly meals on a regular basis, lowering the risk of symptom flare-ups including bloating, stomach discomfort, and diarrhea.

2. ****Nutritional Absorption:**** You can increase the absorption of key vitamins and minerals that may be limited due to SIBO by eating nutrient-dense foods and properly planning meals.

3. **Consistent Energy Levels:** Balanced meals may help maintain consistent energy levels throughout the day, minimizing weariness and lethargy that are often linked with SIBO.

4. **Gut Health Support:** Proper meal planning supports gut health by reducing irritants and offering healthy, easy-to-digest meals that aid in intestinal lining mending.

5. **Customization:** Meal planning enables you to personalize your diet to your unique sensitivities and interests while remaining true to SIBO dietary guidelines.

6. **Reduced Stress:** Planning your meals ahead of time minimizes mealtime stress and allows you to make more conscious choices that match with your nutritional objectives.

7. **Compliance and Consistency:** Following a SIBO diet consistently via meal planning enhances adherence to dietary restrictions, resulting in more effective symptom management and better gut health.

8. **Weight Control:** Meal planning may help you maintain a healthy weight, which can be difficult for some people with SIBO owing to malabsorption concerns.

9. **Long-Term Success:** Effective meal planning lays the groundwork for long-term SIBO treatment, allowing you to retain dietary control even after symptoms have subsided.

10. **Progress Reporting:** As part of your meal planning process, keep a meal diary to track how various foods and meal combinations influence your symptoms, allowing you to fine-tune your diet over time.

Finally, meal planning for a SIBO diet is a proactive strategy to symptom relief and gut health support. Individuals with SIBO may benefit from better symptom management, greater nutrient absorption, and long-term success in controlling their illness by carefully choosing meals, balancing macronutrients, and following to dietary recommendations. Consultation with a healthcare physician or registered dietitian who is familiar with SIBO treatment may give tailored advice and improve the efficacy of your meal planning efforts.

14-days Meal Plan

Day 1:

Breakfast:
- Scrambled eggs with spinach and tomatoes
- Sliced kiwi

Lunch:
- Grilled chicken breast with quinoa
- Steamed carrots and green beans

Snack:
- Almonds (a small portion)

Dinner:
- Baked salmon with lemon and dill
- Mashed potatoes (made with lactose-free milk and olive oil)
- Roasted zucchini

Day 2:

Breakfast:

- Greek yogurt (lactose-free) with blueberries and a drizzle of honey (if tolerated)

Lunch:
- Quinoa salad with cucumber, bell peppers, and grilled shrimp
- Lemon vinaigrette dressing

Snack:
- Sliced cantaloupe

Dinner:
- Turkey meatballs with homemade tomato sauce (no onion or garlic)
- Steamed broccoli
- Brown rice (small portion)

Day 3:
Breakfast:
- Smoothie with lactose-free yogurt, banana, and spinach

Lunch:
- Spinach and grilled chicken salad with a low-FODMAP dressing

Snack:
- Rice cakes with almond butter (in moderation)

Dinner:
- Baked cod with a side of quinoa and sautéed spinach

Day 4:

Breakfast:
- Omelette with tomatoes, green bell peppers, and cheddar cheese (lactose-free)

Lunch:
- Turkey and avocado lettuce wraps with a side of carrot sticks

Snack:
- Fresh raspberries

Dinner:
- Stir-fried tofu with bok choy, ginger, and gluten-free soy sauce
- Steamed jasmine rice (small portion)

Day 5:

Breakfast:

- Overnight oats made with gluten-free oats, chia seeds, almond milk, and topped with strawberries

Lunch:
- Grilled shrimp and quinoa bowl with mixed greens and a lemon-tahini dressing

Snack:
- Baby carrots with hummus (in moderation)

Dinner:
- Baked chicken thighs with rosemary and roasted sweet potatoes
- Steamed green beans

Day 6:

Breakfast:
- Scrambled eggs with spinach and lactose-free cheddar cheese

Lunch:
- Spinach and arugula salad with grilled salmon and a citrus vinaigrette

Snack:
- Sliced kiwi

Dinner:
- Beef and vegetable stir-fry with gluten-free soy sauce
- Jasmine rice (small portion)

Day 7:

Breakfast:
- Smoothie with lactose-free yogurt, banana, and frozen blueberries

Lunch:
- Turkey and quinoa stuffed bell peppers (no onion or garlic)

Snack:
- Almonds (a small portion)

Dinner:
- Baked trout with lemon and fresh herbs
- Mashed potatoes (made with lactose-free milk and olive oil)
- Sautéed asparagus

Day 8:

Breakfast:

- Greek yogurt (lactose-free) with raspberries and a drizzle of honey (if tolerated)

Lunch:
- Grilled chicken salad with mixed greens, cherry tomatoes, and a low-FODMAP dressing

Snack:
- Sliced cantaloupe

Dinner:
- Pork tenderloin with a side of quinoa and steamed broccoli

Day 9:

Breakfast:
- Omelette with spinach, tomatoes, and lactose-free cheddar cheese

Lunch:
- Tuna salad (made with lactose-free mayo) on lettuce leaves

Snack:
- Rice cakes with almond butter (in moderation)

Dinner:

- Baked cod with a side of brown rice and sautéed zucchini

Day 10:

Breakfast:
- Overnight oats made with gluten-free oats, chia seeds, almond milk, and topped with sliced banana (if tolerated)

Lunch:
- Quinoa and mixed greens salad with grilled shrimp and a lemon-tahini dressing

Snack:
- Baby carrots with hummus (in moderation)

Dinner:
- Chicken and vegetable stir-fry with gluten-free soy sauce
- Steamed jasmine rice (small portion)

Day 11:

Breakfast:
- Scrambled eggs with spinach and lactose-free cheddar cheese

Lunch:
- Spinach and arugula salad with grilled salmon and a citrus vinaigrette

Snack:
- Sliced kiwi

Dinner:
- Beef and broccoli stir-fry with gluten-free soy sauce
- Steamed jasmine rice (small portion)

Day 12:

Breakfast:
- Smoothie with lactose-free yogurt, banana, and frozen strawberries

Lunch:
- Turkey and quinoa stuffed bell peppers (no onion or garlic)

Snack:
- Almonds (a small portion)

Dinner:
- Baked trout with lemon and fresh herbs

- Mashed potatoes (made with lactose-free milk and olive oil)
- Sautéed asparagus

Day 13:

Breakfast:
- Greek yogurt (lactose-free) with blueberries and a drizzle of honey (if tolerated)

Lunch:
- Grilled chicken salad with mixed greens, cherry tomatoes, and a low-FODMAP dressing

Snack:
- Sliced cantaloupe

Dinner:
- Pork tenderloin with a side of quinoa and steamed broccoli

Day 14:

Breakfast:
- Omelette with spinach, tomatoes, and lactose-free cheddar cheese

Lunch:

- Tuna salad (made with lactose-free mayo) on lettuce leaves

Snack:
- Rice cakes with almond butter (in moderation)

Dinner:
- Baked cod with a side of brown rice and sautéed zucchini

Remember to stay hydrated throughout the day by drinking plenty of water or herbal teas. This sample meal plan provides a variety of SIBO-friendly options to help manage symptoms and support your overall well-being. Adjust portion sizes and ingredients based on your individual tolerance and preferences.

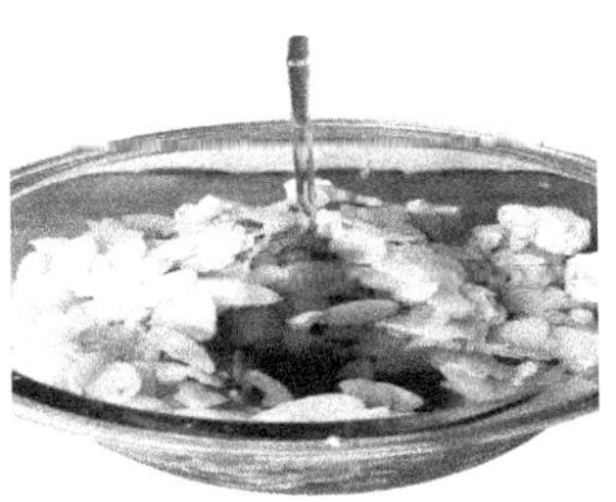

Chapter 5
SIBO-Friendly Recipes

Breakfast Recipes

1. Scrambled Eggs with Spinach and Tomatoes:

Ingredients:
- 2 large eggs
- 1/2 cup fresh spinach
- 1/2 cup diced tomatoes
- Salt and pepper to taste
- 1 teaspoon olive oil

Preparation:
1. In a bowl, whisk the eggs, salt, and pepper.
2. Heat olive oil in a non-stick pan over medium heat.
3. Add spinach and tomatoes, sauté for 2 minutes.
4. Pour in the egg mixture and scramble until cooked through (about 3-4 minutes).

Quantity: 1 serving

Nutritional Value (approx.):
- Calories: 240
- Protein: 14g
- Carbohydrates: 7g
- Fat: 18g
- Fiber: 2g

Cooking Time: 10 minutes

2. Greek Yogurt with Berries:

Ingredients:
- 1 cup lactose-free Greek yogurt
- 1/2 cup mixed berries (e.g., blueberries, strawberries)
- 1 tablespoon honey (if tolerated)

Preparation:
1. Spoon Greek yogurt into a bowl.
2. Wash and slice your berries
3. Top with mixed berries and drizzle with honey.

Quantity: 1 serving

Nutritional Value (approx.):
- Calories: 200

- Protein: 15g
- Carbohydrates: 30g
- Fat: 2g
- Fiber: 4g

Cooking Time: 5 minutes (assembly)

3. Smoothie with Spinach and Banana:

Ingredients:
- 1 cup lactose-free yogurt
- 1 ripe banana (if tolerated)
- 1 cup fresh spinach
- 1/2 cup almond milk
- 1 tablespoon chia seeds

Preparation:
1. Blend all ingredients until smooth.

Quantity: 1 serving

Nutritional Value (approx.):
- Calories: 280
- Protein: 10g

- Carbohydrates: 45g
- Fat: 8g
- Fiber: 10g

Cooking Time: 5 minutes

4. Omelette with Spinach and Lactose-Free Cheddar:

Ingredients:
- 2 large eggs
- 1/2 cup fresh spinach
- 1/4 cup lactose-free cheddar cheese, shredded
- Salt and pepper to taste
- 1 teaspoon olive oil

Preparation:
1. In a bowl, whisk the eggs, salt, and pepper.
2. Heat olive oil in a non-stick pan over medium heat.
3. Add spinach and sauté for 2 minutes.
4. Pour in the egg mixture, sprinkle with cheddar, and cook until set (about 3-4 minutes).

Quantity: 1 serving

Nutritional Value (approx.):
- Calories: 310
- Protein: 21g
- Carbohydrates: 3g
- Fat: 24g
- Fiber: 1g

Cooking Time: 10 minutes

5. Overnight Oats with Blueberries:

Ingredients:
- 1/2 cup gluten-free oats
- 1 tablespoon chia seeds
- 1 cup almond milk
- 1/2 cup fresh blueberries
- 1 teaspoon maple syrup (if tolerated)

Preparation:
1. Mix oats, chia seeds, almond milk, and maple syrup (if using) in a jar.
2. Seal and refrigerate overnight.
3. In the morning, top with fresh blueberries.
4. Serve immediately.

Quantity: 1 serving

Nutritional Value (approx.):
- Calories: 300
- Protein: 8g
- Carbohydrates: 48g
- Fat: 8g
- Fiber: 11g

Cooking Time: Overnight (no cooking)

6. Almond Butter and Banana Rice Cakes:

Ingredients:
- 2 rice cakes (gluten-free)
- 2 tablespoons almond butter
- 1 small ripe banana (if tolerated)

Preparation:
1. Spread almond butter on rice cakes.
2. Top with banana slices.

Quantity: 1 serving

Nutritional Value (approx.):
- Calories: 320
- Protein: 7g
- Carbohydrates: 40g
- Fat: 16g
- Fiber: 4g

Cooking Time: 2 minutes (assembly)

7. Lactose-Free Yogurt Parfait:

Ingredients:
- 1 cup lactose-free yogurt
- 1/4 cup gluten-free granola
- 1/2 cup mixed berries
- 1 teaspoon honey (if tolerated)

Preparation:
1. Layer yogurt, granola, mixed berries, and drizzle with honey (if using) in a glass or bowl.

Quantity: 1 serving

Nutritional Value (approx.):
- Calories: 290

- Protein: 10g
- Carbohydrates: 45g
- Fat: 8g
- Fiber: 5g

Cooking Time: 5 minutes (assembly)

8. Spinach and Tomato Frittata:

Ingredients:
- 4 large eggs
- 1/2 cup fresh spinach
- 1/2 cup diced tomatoes
- Salt and pepper to taste
- 1 teaspoon olive oil

Preparation:
1. In a bowl, whisk the eggs, salt, and pepper.
2. Heat olive oil in an oven-safe pan over medium heat.
3. Add spinach and tomatoes, sauté for 2 minutes.
4. Pour in the egg mixture and cook for 2-3 minutes. Finish cooking under the broiler for an additional 2 minutes.

Quantity: 1 serving

Nutritional Value (approx.):
- Calories: 240
- Protein: 15g
- Carbohydrates: 5g
- Fat: 18g
- Fiber: 2g

Cooking Time: 10 minutes

9. Quinoa and Mixed Berry Breakfast Bowl:

Ingredients:
- 1/2 cup cooked quinoa
- 1/2 cup mixed berries (e.g., blueberries, raspberries)
- 1 tablespoon chia seeds
- 1 tablespoon almond slivers
- 1 teaspoon honey (if tolerated)

Preparation:
1. In a bowl, combine cooked quinoa, mixed berries, chia seeds, and almond slivers.
2. Drizzle with honey (if using).

Quantity: 1 serving

Nutritional Value (approx.):
- Calories: 300
- Protein: 6g
- Carbohydrates: 50g
- Fat: 7g
- Fiber: 8g

Cooking Time: 15 minutes (including quinoa preparation)

10. Banana and Almond Milk Smoothie:

Ingredients:
- 1 ripe banana (if tolerated)
- 1 cup almond milk
- 1 tablespoon almond butter
- 1 teaspoon chia seeds

Preparation:
1. Blend ripe banana, almond milk, almond butter, and chia seeds until smooth.

Quantity: 1 serving

Nutritional Value (approx.):
- Calories: 260
- Protein: 3g
- Carbohydrates: 30g
- Fat: 14g
- Fiber: 6g

Cooking Time: 5 minutes

These SIBO-friendly breakfast recipes offer a variety of flavors and textures while adhering to dietary principles. Adjust quantities and ingredients based on your specific dietary tolerances and preferences. These meals are designed to be easy to prepare and nutritious, supporting your SIBO management plan while providing a satisfying start to your day.

Lunch Recipes

1. Grilled Chicken Salad with Lemon-Tahini Dressing:

Ingredients:
- 4 oz grilled chicken breast

- 2 cups mixed greens
- 1/4 cup cucumber slices
- 1/4 cup cherry tomatoes
- 2 tablespoons lemon-tahini dressing (made with tahini, lemon juice, olive oil, and salt)

Preparation:
1. Grill the chicken until fully cooked and slice it.
2. Assemble mixed greens, cucumber slices, cherry tomatoes, and grilled chicken in a bowl.
3. Drizzle with lemon-tahini dressing.

Quantity: 1 serving

Nutritional Value (approx.):
- Calories: 320
- Protein: 30g
- Carbohydrates: 10g
- Fat: 18g
- Fiber: 3g

Cooking Time: 15 minutes

2. Quinoa and Mixed Veggie Bowl:

Ingredients:
- 1 cup cooked quinoa
- 1/2 cup steamed carrots
- 1/2 cup steamed green beans
- 1/4 cup diced red bell pepper
- 2 tablespoons olive oil
- 1 tablespoon fresh lemon juice
- Salt and pepper to taste

Preparation:
1. Cook quinoa according to package instructions.
2. Steam carrots and green beans until tender.
3. Toss quinoa, steamed vegetables, red bell pepper, olive oil, lemon juice, salt, and pepper in a bowl.

Quantity: 1 serving

Nutritional Value (approx.):
- Calories: 380
- Protein: 8g
- Carbohydrates: 40g
- Fat: 22g
- Fiber: 7g

Cooking Time: 20 minutes

3. Tuna Salad Lettuce Wraps:

Ingredients:
- 1 can (5 oz) tuna, drained
- 2 tablespoons lactose-free mayonnaise
- 1/4 cup diced celery
- 1/4 cup diced cucumber
- 4 large lettuce leaves (e.g., iceberg or romaine)

Preparation:
1. In a bowl, mix tuna, lactose-free mayonnaise, celery, and cucumber.
2. Spoon the tuna salad onto lettuce leaves and wrap them.

Quantity: 1 serving

Nutritional Value (approx.):
- Calories: 240
- Protein: 22g
- Carbohydrates: 3g
- Fat: 15g
- Fiber: 1g

Cooking Time: 10 minutes

4. Turkey and Quinoa Stuffed Bell Peppers:

Ingredients:

- 2 large bell peppers
- 1/2 cup cooked quinoa
- 4 oz ground turkey
- 1/4 cup diced tomatoes
- 1/4 cup diced zucchini
- 1/4 cup diced carrots
- Salt and pepper to taste

Preparation:

1. Preheat the oven to 375°F (190°C).
2. Cut the tops off the bell peppers and remove seeds.
3. In a skillet, cook ground turkey until browned. Add diced vegetables and cook until tender.
4. Stir in cooked quinoa, salt, and pepper.
5. Stuff the bell peppers with the turkey and quinoa mixture.
6. Place stuffed peppers in a baking dish, cover with foil, and bake for 25-30 minutes until peppers are tender.

Quantity: 2 servings (1/2 stuffed pepper per serving)

Nutritional Value (approx. per serving):
- Calories: 220
- Protein: 18g
- Carbohydrates: 18g
- Fat: 8g
- Fiber: 4g

Cooking Time: 50 minutes (including baking)

5. Spinach and Grilled Salmon Salad:

Ingredients:
- 4 oz grilled salmon
- 2 cups fresh spinach
- 1/4 cup sliced strawberries
- 1/4 cup sliced almonds
- 2 tablespoons balsamic vinaigrette (low-FODMAP)

Preparation:
1. Grill salmon until fully cooked and flaky.
2. Assemble spinach, sliced strawberries, grilled salmon, and sliced almonds in a bowl.
3. Drizzle with balsamic vinaigrette.

Quantity: 1 serving

Nutritional Value (approx.):
- Calories: 350
- Protein: 28g
- Carbohydrates: 12g
- Fat: 20g
- Fiber: 4g

Cooking Time: 15 minutes

6. Turkey and Avocado Lettuce Wraps:

Ingredients:
- 4 large lettuce leaves
- 4 oz sliced turkey breast
- 1/2 avocado, sliced
- 1/4 cup shredded carrots

- 1/4 cup cucumber slices
- 1 tablespoon olive oil
- 1 tablespoon lemon juice
- Salt and pepper to taste

Preparation:

1. Arrange turkey slices, avocado, shredded carrots, and cucumber on lettuce leaves.
2. Drizzle with olive oil and lemon juice.
3. Season with salt and pepper.

Quantity: 2 servings (2 lettuce wraps per serving)

Nutritional Value (approx. per serving):

- Calories: 270
- Protein: 18g
- Carbohydrates: 10g
- Fat: 20g
- Fiber: 5g

Cooking Time: 10 minutes

7. Chicken and Vegetable Stir-Fry:

Ingredients:
- 4 oz cooked chicken breast, sliced
- 1/2 cup green beans
- 1/2 cup bell peppers (any color), sliced
- 1/2 cup zucchini, sliced
- 2 tablespoons gluten-free soy sauce
- 1 teaspoon fresh ginger, minced
- 1 teaspoon sesame

Preparation:
1. Heat a non-stick skillet or wok over medium-high heat.
2. Add cooked chicken slices and stir-fry for 2 minutes.
3. Add green beans, bell peppers, and zucchini. Continue stir-frying for 5-7 minutes until vegetables are tender.
4. Stir in gluten-free soy sauce and minced ginger. Cook for an additional 2 minutes.

Quantity: 1 serving

Nutritional Value (approx.):
- Calories: 280

- Protein: 35g
- Carbohydrates: 14g
- Fat: 8g
- Fiber: 4g

Cooking Time: 15 minutes

8. Pork Tenderloin with Quinoa and Steamed Broccoli:

Ingredients:
- 4 oz cooked pork tenderloin
- 1/2 cup cooked quinoa
- 1 cup steamed broccoli
- 1 tablespoon olive oil
- 1 tablespoon balsamic vinegar (low-FODMAP)
- Salt and pepper to taste

Preparation:
1. Cook pork tenderloin until fully done.
2. Cook quinoa according to package instructions.
3. Steam broccoli until tender.
4. Slice pork tenderloin and assemble with quinoa and steamed broccoli.

5. Drizzle with olive oil and balsamic vinegar. Season with salt and pepper.

Quantity: 1 serving

Nutritional Value (approx.):
- Calories: 340
- Protein: 32g
- Carbohydrates: 28g
- Fat: 12g
- Fiber: 6g

Cooking Time: 30 minutes (including pork tenderloin and quinoa cooking)

9. Beef and Broccoli Stir-Fry:

Ingredients:
- 4 oz lean beef (e.g., sirloin), sliced
- 1 cup broccoli florets
- 2 tablespoons gluten-free soy sauce
- 1 teaspoon fresh ginger, minced
- 1 teaspoon sesame oil
- 1/2 cup cooked brown rice

Preparation:
1. Heat a non-stick skillet or wok over medium-high heat.
2. Add sliced beef and stir-fry for 2 minutes.
3. Add broccoli florets and continue stir-frying for 5-7 minutes until beef is cooked and broccoli is tender.
4. Stir in gluten-free soy sauce, minced ginger, and sesame oil. Cook for an additional 2 minutes.
5. Serve over cooked brown rice.

Quantity: 1 serving

Nutritional Value (approx.):
- Calories: 350
- Protein: 30g
- Carbohydrates: 30g
- Fat: 12g
- Fiber: 5g

Cooking Time: 20 minutes

10. Baked Cod with Brown Rice and Sautéed Zucchini:

Ingredients:

- 4 oz cod fillet
- 1/2 cup cooked brown rice
- 1 cup sliced zucchini
- 1 tablespoon olive oil
- 1 teaspoon fresh lemon juice
- Salt and pepper to taste

Preparation:

1. Preheat the oven to 375°F (190°C).
2. Place cod fillet on a baking sheet, drizzle with olive oil and lemon juice, and season with salt and pepper.
3. Bake for 15-20 minutes until cod is opaque and flakes easily.
4. While the cod is baking, sauté sliced zucchini in a pan with olive oil until tender.
5. Serve baked cod with brown rice and sautéed zucchini.

Quantity: 1 serving

Nutritional Value (approx.):

- Calories: 310
- Protein: 30g
- Carbohydrates: 35g
- Fat: 8g
- Fiber: 5g

Cooking Time: 25 minutes (including cod baking)

These SIBO-friendly lunch recipes offer a variety of flavors and textures while adhering to dietary principles. Adjust quantities and ingredients based on your specific dietary tolerances and preferences. These meals are designed to be easy to prepare and nutritious, supporting your SIBO management plan during lunchtime.

Dinner Recipes

1. Baked Salmon with Lemon and Dill:

Ingredients:
- 6 oz salmon fillet
- 1 tablespoon fresh lemon juice
- 1 teaspoon dried dill
- Salt and pepper to taste

Preparation:
1. Preheat the oven to 375°F (190°C).

2. Place salmon fillet on a baking sheet, drizzle with lemon juice, sprinkle with dried dill, salt, and pepper.

3. Bake for 15-20 minutes until salmon flakes easily with a fork.

Quantity: 1 serving

Nutritional Value (approx.):
- Calories: 300
- Protein: 35g
- Carbohydrates: 0g
- Fat: 18g
- Fiber: 0g

Cooking Time: 20 minutes

2. Grilled Chicken with Quinoa and Roasted Vegetables:

Ingredients:
- 4 oz grilled chicken breast
- 1/2 cup cooked quinoa

- 1 cup mixed roasted vegetables (e.g., bell peppers, zucchini, carrots)
- 1 tablespoon olive oil
- Salt and pepper to taste

Preparation:
1. Grill chicken until fully cooked and slice it.
2. Cook quinoa according to package instructions.
3. Toss roasted vegetables with olive oil, salt, and pepper.
4. Assemble grilled chicken, cooked quinoa, and roasted vegetables on a plate.

Quantity: 1 serving

Nutritional Value (approx.):
- Calories: 350
- Protein: 30g
- Carbohydrates: 30g
- Fat: 12g
- Fiber: 6g

Cooking Time: 30 minutes (including grilling and roasting)

3. Stir-Fried Tofu with Bok Choy and Ginger:

Ingredients:
- 6 oz firm tofu, cubed
- 1 cup chopped bok choy
- 1 teaspoon fresh ginger, minced
- 2 tablespoons gluten-free soy sauce
- 1 tablespoon sesame oil
- 1/2 cup cooked jasmine rice

Preparation:
1. Heat a non-stick skillet or wok over medium-high heat.
2. Add cubed tofu and stir-fry until lightly browned.
3. Add chopped bok choy and minced ginger. Continue stir-frying for 3-4 minutes.
4. Stir in gluten-free soy sauce and sesame oil. Cook for an additional 2 minutes.
5. Serve over cooked jasmine rice.

Quantity: 1 serving

Nutritional Value (approx.):
- Calories: 380
- Protein: 14g
- Carbohydrates: 45g

- Fat: 18g
- Fiber: 5g

Cooking Time: 20 minutes

4. Baked Cod with a Side of Brown Rice and Sautéed Zucchini:

Ingredients:
- 6 oz cod fillet
- 1/2 cup cooked brown rice
- 1 cup sliced zucchini
- 1 tablespoon olive oil
- 1 teaspoon fresh lemon juice
- Salt and pepper to taste

Preparation:
1. Preheat the oven to 375°F (190°C).
2. Place cod fillet on a baking sheet, drizzle with olive oil and lemon juice, and season with salt and pepper.
3. Bake for 15-20 minutes until cod is opaque and flakes easily.
4. While the cod is baking, sauté sliced zucchini in a pan with olive oil until tender.

5. Serve baked cod with brown rice and sautéed zucchini.

Quantity: 1 serving

Nutritional Value (approx.):
- Calories: 340
- Protein: 30g
- Carbohydrates: 35g
- Fat: 8g
- Fiber: 5g

Cooking Time: 25 minutes (including cod baking)

5. Turkey Meatballs with Homemade Tomato Sauce:

Ingredients:
- 4 turkey meatballs (homemade, no onion or garlic)
- 1/2 cup tomato sauce (homemade, no onion or garlic)
- 1/2 cup cooked gluten-free pasta (e.g., rice pasta)

Preparation:

1. Prepare turkey meatballs and tomato sauce following SIBO-friendly recipes.
2. Cook gluten-free pasta according to package instructions.
3. Serve turkey meatballs with tomato sauce over cooked pasta.

Quantity: 1 serving

Nutritional Value (approx.):
- Calories: 380
- Protein: 30g
- Carbohydrates: 40g
- Fat: 10g
- Fiber: 3g

Cooking Time: Varies (depending on meatball and sauce preparation)

6. Pork Tenderloin with Quinoa and Steamed Broccoli:

Ingredients:
- 4 oz cooked pork tenderloin

- 1/2 cup cooked quinoa
- 1 cup steamed broccoli
- 1 tablespoon olive oil
- 1 tablespoon balsamic vinegar (low-FODMAP)
- Salt and pepper to taste

Preparation:
1. Cook pork tenderloin until fully done.
2. Cook quinoa according to package instructions.
3. Steam broccoli until tender.
4. Slice pork tenderloin and assemble with quinoa and steamed broccoli.
5. Drizzle with olive oil and balsamic vinegar. Season with salt and pepper.

Quantity: 1 serving

Nutritional Value (approx.):
- Calories: 340
- Protein: 30g
- Carbohydrates: 28g
- Fat: 12g
- Fiber: 6g

Cooking Time:** 30 minutes (including pork tenderloin and quinoa cooking)

7. Beef and Broccoli Stir-Fry:

Ingredients:
- 4 oz lean beef (e.g., sirloin), sliced
- 1 cup broccoli florets
- 2 tablespoons gluten-free soy sauce
- 1 teaspoon fresh ginger, minced
- 1 teaspoon sesame oil
- 1/2 cup cooked brown rice

Preparation:
1. Heat a non-stick skillet or wok over medium-high heat.
2. Add sliced beef and stir-fry for 2 minutes.
3. Add broccoli florets and continue stir-frying for 5-7 minutes until beef is cooked and broccoli is tender.
4. Stir in gluten-free soy sauce, minced ginger, and sesame oil. Cook for an additional 2 minutes.
5. Serve over cooked brown rice.

Quantity: 1 serving

Nutritional Value (approx.):
- Calories: 350

- Protein: 30g
- Carbohydrates: 30g
- Fat: 12g
- Fiber: 5g

Cooking Time: 20 minutes

8. Spinach and Tomato Stuffed Chicken Breast:

Ingredients:
- 6 oz chicken breast
- 1/4 cup fresh spinach leaves
- 1/4 cup diced tomatoes (canned, no onion or garlic)
- 1 tablespoon olive oil
- 1 teaspoon dried basil
- Salt and pepper to taste

Preparation:
1. Preheat the oven to 375°F (190°C).
2. Slice a pocket into the side of the chicken breast.
3. Stuff the pocket with fresh spinach and diced tomatoes.
4. Drizzle olive oil over the chicken, sprinkle with dried basil, salt, and pepper.

5. Bake for 25-30 minutes until the chicken is cooked through.

Quantity: 1 serving

Nutritional Value (approx.):
- Calories: 280
- Protein: 30g
- Carbohydrates: 4g
- Fat: 16g
- Fiber: 2g

Cooking Time: 30 minutes (including baking)

9. Shrimp and Zucchini Noodles with Pesto:

Ingredients:
- 4 oz cooked shrimp (peeled and deveined)
- 1 large zucchini, spiralized into noodles
- 2 tablespoons homemade pesto sauce (made without garlic)
- 1 tablespoon grated Parmesan cheese (optional)

Preparation:

1. Cook shrimp until pink and opaque.
2. Spiralize zucchini into noodles using a spiralizer or julienne peeler.
3. Toss zucchini noodles with homemade pesto sauce.
4. Top with cooked shrimp and, if desired, grated Parmesan cheese.

Quantity: 1 serving

Nutritional Value (approx.):
- Calories: 320
- Protein: 30g
- Carbohydrates: 10g
- Fat: 18g
- Fiber: 3g

Cooking Time: 15 minutes (including shrimp cooking)

10. Lemon Herb Baked Chicken Thighs:

Ingredients:
- 2 boneless, skinless chicken thighs

- 1 tablespoon fresh lemon juice
- 1 teaspoon dried thyme
- 1 teaspoon dried rosemary
- Salt and pepper to taste

Preparation:
1. Preheat the oven to 375°F (190°C).
2. Place chicken thighs on a baking sheet.
3. Drizzle fresh lemon juice over the chicken, sprinkle with dried thyme, dried rosemary, salt, and pepper.
4. Bake for 25-30 minutes until the chicken is fully cooked.

Quantity: 1 serving

Nutritional Value (approx.):
- Calories: 320
  Protein: 30g
- Carbohydrates: 2g
- Fat: 18g
- Fiber: 0g

Cooking Time: 30 minutes

These SIBO-friendly dinner recipes offer a variety of flavors and textures while adhering to dietary principles. Adjust quantities and ingredients based on your specific dietary tolerances and preferences. These meals are designed to be easy to prepare and nutritious, supporting your SIBO management plan during dinner.

Dessert Recipes

1. Berry Parfait with Lactose-Free Yogurt:

Ingredients:
- 1 cup lactose-free yogurt
- 1/2 cup mixed berries (e.g., blueberries, strawberries)
- 1 tablespoon honey (if tolerated)

Preparation:
1. Layer lactose-free yogurt and mixed berries in a glass or bowl.
2. Drizzle with honey (if using).

Quantity: 1 serving

Nutritional Value (approx.):

- Calories: 220
- Protein: 10g
- Carbohydrates: 30g
- Fat: 7g
- Fiber: 4g

Preparation Time: 5 minutes (assembly)

2. Chocolate Avocado Mousse:

Ingredients:
- 1 ripe avocado
- 2 tablespoons cocoa powder (unsweetened)
- 2 tablespoons maple syrup (if tolerated)
- 1/2 teaspoon vanilla extract

Preparation:
1. Scoop the flesh of the ripe avocado into a blender or food processor.
2. Add cocoa powder, maple syrup (if using), and vanilla extract.
3. Blend until smooth and creamy.
4. Refrigerate for 30 minutes before serving.

Quantity: 1 serving

Nutritional Value (approx.):
- Calories: 250
- Protein: 3g
- Carbohydrates: 28g
- Fat: 17g
- Fiber: 9g

Preparation Time: 10 minutes (plus chilling time)

3. Banana and Almond Butter Bites:

Ingredients:
- 1 ripe banana (if tolerated)
- 2 tablespoons almond butter
- 1 tablespoon unsweetened shredded coconut (optional)

Preparation:
1. Slice the banana into bite-sized rounds.
2. Spread almond butter on each banana slice.

3. Sprinkle with unsweetened shredded coconut if desired.

Quantity: Varies (depending on the size of the banana)

Nutritional Value (approx. per serving):
- Calories: 120
- Protein: 2g
- Carbohydrates: 15g
- Fat: 7g
- Fiber: 3g

Preparation Time: 5 minutes

4. Chia Seed Pudding with Berries:

Ingredients:
- 2 tablespoons chia seeds
- 1 cup almond milk
- 1/2 cup mixed berries (e.g., raspberries, blackberries)
- 1 teaspoon honey (if tolerated)

Preparation:

1. In a bowl, mix chia seeds and almond milk. Stir well.
2. Refrigerate for at least 2 hours or overnight, stirring occasionally to prevent clumping.
3. Before serving, top with mixed berries and drizzle with honey (if using).

Quantity: 1 serving

Nutritional Value (approx.):
- Calories: 190
- Protein: 4g
- Carbohydrates: 24g
- Fat: 10g
- Fiber: 11g

Preparation Time: 2 hours or more (including refrigeration)

5. Baked Apples with Cinnamon and Walnuts:

Ingredients:
- 1 medium apple (if tolerated)

- 1/2 teaspoon ground cinnamon
- 1 tablespoon chopped walnuts
- 1 teaspoon honey (if tolerated)

Preparation:

1. Preheat the oven to 350°F (180°C).
2. Core the apple and place it in an oven-safe dish.
3. Sprinkle with ground cinnamon and stuff with chopped walnuts.
4. Drizzle with honey (if using).
5. Bake for 25-30 minutes until the apple is tender.

Quantity: 1 serving

Nutritional Value (approx.):

- Calories: 180
- Protein: 2g
- Carbohydrates: 28g
- Fat: 8g
- Fiber: 5g

Cooking Time: 30 minutes

6. Coconut Rice Pudding:

Ingredients:

- 1/2 cup cooked glutinous rice (sticky rice)
- 1/2 cup coconut milk (unsweetened)
- 1 tablespoon maple syrup (if tolerated)
- 1/2 teaspoon vanilla extract

Preparation:

1. In a saucepan, combine cooked glutinous rice, coconut milk, maple syrup (if using), and vanilla extract.
2. Heat over low-medium heat, stirring continuously until it thickens (about 10-15 minutes).
3. Remove from heat and let it cool before serving.

Quantity: 1 serving

Nutritional Value (approx.):
- Calories: 350
- Protein: 3g
- Carbohydrates: 38g
- Fat: 22g
- Fiber: 2g

Cooking Time: 15 minutes

7. Mixed Berry Sorbet:

Ingredients:
- 1 cup mixed berries (e.g., strawberries, blueberries)
- 2 tablespoons fresh lemon juice
- 1 tablespoon maple syrup (if tolerated)

Preparation:
1. Place mixed berries, fresh lemon juice, and maple syrup (if using) in a blender.
2. Blend until smooth.
3. Pour the mixture into a shallow container and freeze for at least 3 hours, stirring every hour to prevent ice crystals.
4. Scoop and serve when it reaches a sorbet-like consistency.

Quantity: 1 serving

Nutritional Value (approx.):
- Calories: 110
- Protein: 1g
- Carbohydrates: 28g
- Fat: 0g

Snacks Recipes

1. Cucumber and Hummus Slices:

Ingredients:
- 1 cucumber
- 2 tablespoons SIBO-friendly hummus

Preparation:
1. Wash and slice the cucumber.
2. Serve the cucumber slices with hummus for dipping.

Quantity: Varies (depending on the size of the cucumber)

Nutritional Value (approx. per serving):
- Calories: 40
- Protein: 2g
- Carbohydrates: 7g
- Fat: 1g
- Fiber: 2g

Preparation Time: 5 minutes

2. Rice Cakes with Almond Butter and Sliced Banana:

Ingredients:
- 2 rice cakes (SIBO-friendly)
- 2 tablespoons almond butter
- 1/2 banana, sliced

Preparation:
1. Spread almond butter on the rice cakes.
2. Top with sliced banana.

Quantity: 1 serving

Nutritional Value (approx. per serving):
- Calories: 220
- Protein: 5g
- Carbohydrates: 30g
- Fat: 10g
- Fiber: 3g

Preparation Time: 5 minutes

3. Greek Yogurt with Berries and Honey:

Ingredients:
- 1 cup lactose-free Greek yogurt
- 1/2 cup mixed berries (e.g., blueberries, raspberries)
- 1 teaspoon honey (if tolerated)

Preparation:
1. Spoon Greek yogurt into a bowl.
2. Top with mixed berries and drizzle with honey (if using).

Quantity: 1 serving

Nutritional Value (approx. per serving):
- Calories: 220
- Protein: 15g
- Carbohydrates: 30g
- Fat: 6g
- Fiber: 4g

Preparation Time: 5 minutes

4. Sliced Apple with Almond Butter:

Ingredients:
- 1 medium apple (if tolerated)
- 2 tablespoons almond butter

Preparation:
1. Slice the apple into wedges.
2. Serve with almond butter for dipping.

Quantity: 1 serving

Nutritional Value (approx. per serving):
- Calories: 220
- Protein: 4g
- Carbohydrates: 30g
- Fat: 10g
- Fiber: 6g

Preparation Time: 5 minutes

5. Carrot Sticks with SIBO-Friendly Ranch Dip:

Ingredients:
- 2 carrots, peeled and sliced into sticks
- 1/4 cup SIBO-friendly ranch dip (homemade or store-bought)

Preparation:
1. Wash, peel, and slice the carrots into sticks.
2. Serve with SIBO-friendly ranch dip for dipping.

Quantity: 1 serving

Nutritional Value (approx. per serving):
- Calories: 80
- Protein: 1g
- Carbohydrates: 10g
- Fat: 4g
- Fiber: 3g

Preparation Time: 10 minutes

6. Mixed Nuts and Seeds:

Ingredients:
- 1/4 cup mixed nuts (e.g., almonds, walnuts)
- 1 tablespoon mixed seeds (e.g., pumpkin seeds, sunflower seeds)

**Preparation:
1. Measure out the mixed nuts and seeds.
2. Combine them in a small bowl.

Quantity: 1 serving

Nutritional Value (approx. per serving):
- Calories: 220
- Protein: 7g
- Carbohydrates: 6g
- Fat: 19g
- Fiber: 3g

Preparation Time: 2 minutes

7. Sliced Bell Peppers with Guacamole:

Ingredients:
- 1 bell pepper (red, yellow, or green)
- 1/4 cup SIBO-friendly guacamole (homemade or store-bought)

Preparation:
1. Wash and slice the bell pepper into strips.
2. Serve with SIBO-friendly guacamole for dipping.

Quantity: 1 serving

Nutritional Value (approx. per serving):
- Calories: 120
- Protein: 2g
- Carbohydrates: 10g
- Fat: 8g
- Fiber: 4g

Preparation Time: 5 minutes

These SIBO-friendly snack recipes offer a variety of flavors and textures while adhering to dietary principles. Adjust quantities and ingredients based on your specific dietary tolerances and preferences. These snacks are designed to be easy to prepare and satisfying between meals.

Smoothies Recipes

1. Berry Blast Smoothie:

Ingredients:
- 1/2 cup mixed berries (e.g., blueberries, raspberries)
- 1/2 banana (if tolerated)
- 1/2 cup lactose-free yogurt
- 1/2 cup unsweetened almond milk
- 1 tablespoon chia seeds
- 1 teaspoon honey (if tolerated)

Preparation:
1. Place mixed berries, banana (if using), lactose-free yogurt, almond milk, chia seeds, and honey (if using) in a blender.
2. Blend until smooth.

Quantity: 1 serving

Nutritional Value (approx. per serving):
- Calories: 250

- Protein: 7g
- Carbohydrates: 38g
- Fat: 8g
- Fiber: 9g

Preparation Time: 5 minutes

2. Green Goodness Smoothie:

Ingredients:
- 1 cup spinach leaves
- 1/2 cucumber (if tolerated)
- 1/2 cup pineapple chunks (fresh or canned in juice)
- 1/2 cup coconut water
- 1 tablespoon fresh lime juice
- Ice cubes (optional)

Preparation:
1. Place spinach leaves, cucumber (if using), pineapple chunks, coconut water, and fresh lime juice in a blender.
2. Add ice cubes if you prefer a colder smoothie.
3. Blend until smooth.

Quantity: 1 serving

Nutritional Value (approx. per serving):

- Calories: 130
- Protein: 3g
- Carbohydrates: 32g
- Fat: 1g
- Fiber: 5g

Preparation Time: 5 minutes

3. Creamy Avocado and Cucumber Smoothie:

Ingredients:

- 1/2 ripe avocado
- 1/2 cucumber (if tolerated)
- 1/2 cup lactose-free yogurt
- 1/2 cup unsweetened almond milk
- 1 tablespoon fresh lemon juice
- Ice cubes (optional)

Preparation:

1. Scoop the flesh of the ripe avocado into a blender.

2. Add cucumber (if using), lactose-free yogurt, almond milk, and fresh lemon juice.
3. Add ice cubes if desired.
4. Blend until smooth.

Quantity: 1 serving

Nutritional Value (approx. per serving):
- Calories: 220
- Protein: 6g
- Carbohydrates: 18g
- Fat: 14g
- Fiber: 8g

Preparation Time: 5 minutes

4. Tropical Paradise Smoothie:

Ingredients:
- 1/2 cup fresh or frozen pineapple chunks
- 1/2 cup fresh or frozen mango chunks
- 1/2 cup coconut water
- 1/2 cup unsweetened almond milk
- 1 tablespoon shredded coconut (unsweetened)

Preparation:

1. Place pineapple chunks, mango chunks, coconut water, unsweetened almond milk, and shredded coconut in a blender.
2. Blend until smooth.

Quantity: 1 serving

Nutritional Value (approx. per serving):

- Calories: 180
- Protein: 2g
- Carbohydrates: 40g
- Fat: 4g
- Fiber: 5g

Preparation Time: 5 minutes

5. Banana and Spinach Power Smoothie:

Ingredients:

- 1 ripe banana (if tolerated)
- 1 cup spinach leaves
- 1/2 cup lactose-free yogurt
- 1/2 cup unsweetened almond milk

- 1 tablespoon almond butter (no added sugars)

Preparation:

1. Slice the ripe banana (if using).
2. Place banana slices, spinach leaves, lactose-free yogurt, unsweetened almond milk, and almond butter in a blender.
3. Blend until smooth.

Quantity: 1 serving

Nutritional Value (approx. per serving):

- Calories: 250
- Protein: 8g
- Carbohydrates: 34g
- Fat: 9g
- Fiber: 6g

Preparation Time: 5 minutes

6. Carrot Cake Smoothie:

Ingredients:

- 1/2 cup cooked and cooled carrots (if tolerated)
- 1/2 cup cooked and cooled zucchini (if tolerated)

- 1/2 cup lactose-free yogurt
- 1/2 cup unsweetened almond milk
- 1 teaspoon ground cinnamon
- 1/2 teaspoon vanilla extract

Preparation:

1. Cook and cool carrots and zucchini (if using).
2. Place cooked carrots, cooked zucchini, lactose-free yogurt, unsweetened almond milk, ground cinnamon, and vanilla extract in a blender.
3. Blend until smooth.

Quantity: 1 serving

Nutritional Value (approx. per serving):

- Calories: 130
- Protein: 5g
- Carbohydrates: 18g
- Fat: 4g
- Fiber: 6g

Preparation Time: 5 minutes

7. Blueberry Almond Protein Smoothie:

Ingredients:
- 1/2 cup frozen blueberries
- 1/2 cup lactose-free yogurt
- 1/2 cup unsweetened almond milk
- 1 tablespoon almond butter (no added sugars)
- 1 scoop SIBO-friendly protein powder (e.g., pea protein)

Preparation:
1. Place frozen blueberries, lactose-free yogurt, unsweetened almond milk, almond butter, and protein powder in a blender.
2. Blend until smooth.

Quantity: 1 serving

Nutritional Value (approx. per serving):
- Calories: 280
- Protein: 25g
- Carbohydrates: 24g
- Fat: 10g
- Fiber: 5g

Preparation Time: 5 minutes

These SIBO-friendly smoothie recipes offer a variety of flavors and nutrients while adhering to dietary principles. Adjust quantities and ingredients based on your specific dietary tolerances and preferences. These smoothies are designed to be quick to prepare and provide a nutritious option for snacks or breakfast.

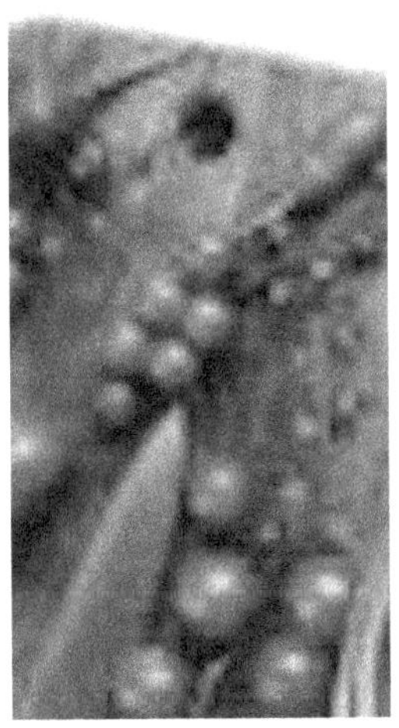

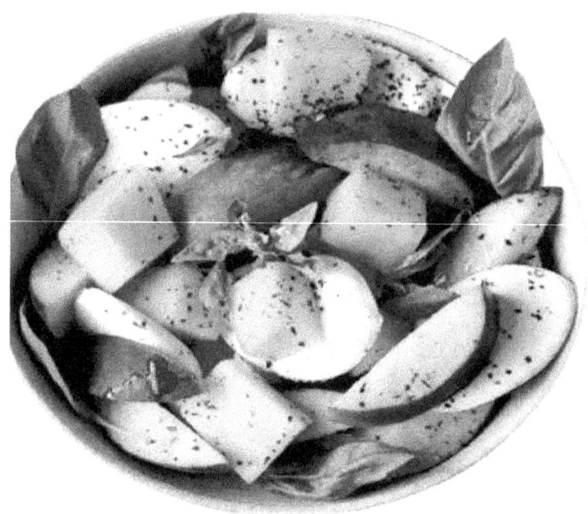

Conclusion

The first step in managing and improving one's quality of life is to understand SIBO (Small Intestinal Bacterial Overgrowth) condition. SIBO is a complicated disorder that may cause a variety of unpleasant symptoms and problems, but it can be properly handled with the appropriate information and approach.

We've examined the definition, kinds, causes, symptoms, and preventative strategies of SIBO throughout this investigation. We've discussed the significance of following a SIBO-friendly diet and the role it plays in symptom relief and general well-being.

A SIBO-friendly diet consists of carefully choosing foods that do not aggravate bacterial overgrowth in the small intestine. Individuals with SIBO may take substantial strides toward treating their illness by avoiding or limiting fermentable carbs, concentrating on low-FODMAP meals, and selecting sources of protein and healthy fats.

The advantages of using a SIBO diet cookbook are many. It not only helps to reduce symptoms and avoid problems, but it also promotes a pleasant connection with food. This cookbook serves as a guide, providing tasty and healthy dishes that demonstrate that treating SIBO does not need losing flavor and pleasure in your meals.

Remember that consistency is essential for individuals commencing on this eating path. Change may not occur immediately, and there may be ups and downs along the road. However, each meal and dish you attempt will get you one step closer to controlling your SIBO and living a better, happier life.

So, my readers, let me leave you with this motivation: Accept the power of food as an ally in the fight against SIBO. Choose foods that are good for you and relish the tastes of each meal. Know that with each meal, you are taking charge of your health and paving the way for a healthier future. Your SIBO management journey may be rewarding, with tasty dishes, better health, and a newfound appreciation for the nutritious possibilities of every food. You have the adaptability, the resilience, and the knowledge to flourish. Your journey to health starts with each mouthful, recipe, and day.

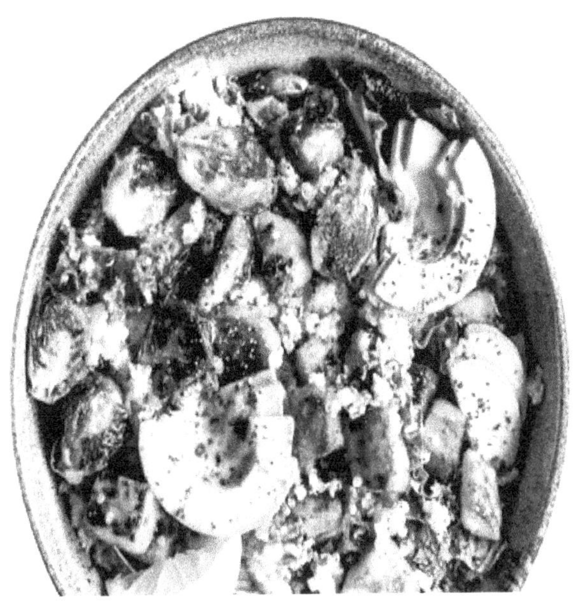

BONUS:

30-Days Meal Planner Journal

SIBO DIET
Daily Meal Planner

Date :

To Do :

M	
T	
W	
Th	
Fri	
Sat	
Sun	

Notes :

Achievement:

Meals :

Breakfast

Lunch

Dinner

Remember, you are not alone. Millions of people around the world suffer from SIBO. But by working together, we can find relief and live our best lives.

Productivity :

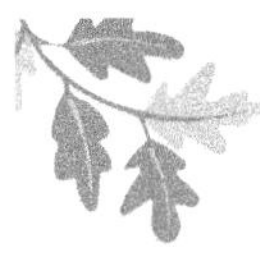

SIBO DIET
Daily Meal Planner

Date :

To Do :

M	
T	
W	
Th	
Fri	
Sat	
Sun	

Notes :

Remember, you are not alone. Millions of people around the world suffer from SIBO. But by working together, we can find relief and live our best lives.

Achievement:

Meals :

Breakfast

Lunch

Dinner

Productivity :

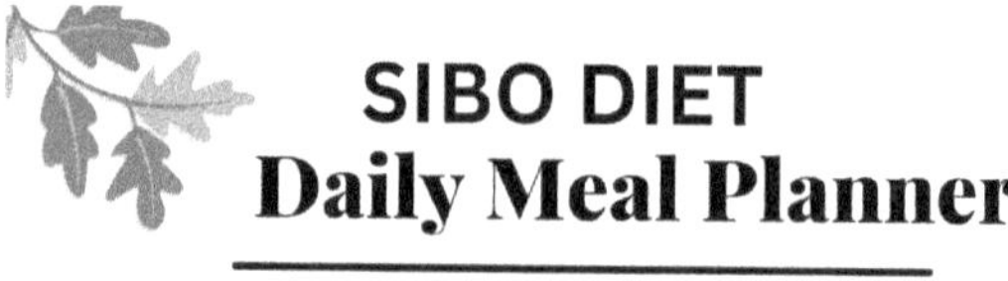

SIBO DIET
Daily Meal Planner

Date :

To Do :

M	
T	
W	
Th	
Fri	
Sat	
Sun	

Notes :

Remember, you are not alone. Millions of people around the world suffer from SIBO. But by working together, we can find relief and live our best lives.

Achievement:

Meals :

Breakfast

Lunch

Dinner

Productivity :

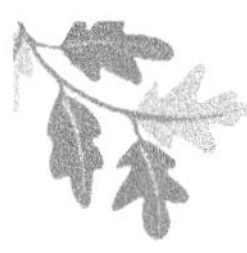

SIBO DIET
Daily Meal Planner

Date :

To Do :

M	
T	
W	
Th	
Fri	
Sat	
Sun	

Notes :

Remember, you are not alone. Millions of people around the world suffer from SIBO. But by working together, we can find relief and live our best lives.

Achievement:

Meals :

Breakfast

Lunch

Dinner

Productivity :

◯ ◯ ◯ ◯ ◯

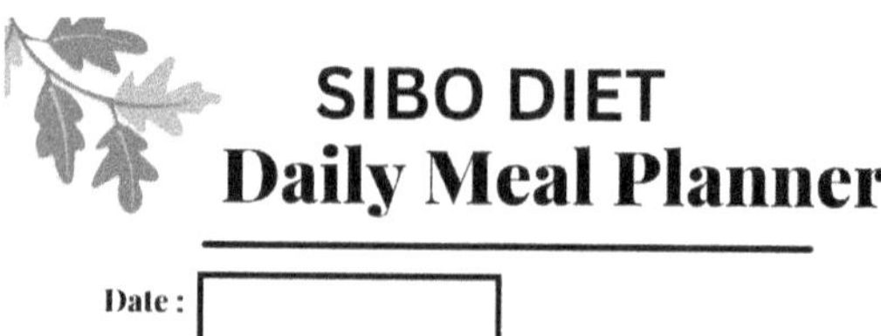

SIBO DIET
Daily Meal Planner

Date :

To Do :

M	
T	
W	
Th	
Fri	
Sat	
Sun	

Notes :

Remember, you are not alone. Millions of people around the world suffer from SIBO. But by working together, we can find relief and live our best lives.

Achievement:

Meals :

Breakfast

Lunch

Dinner

Productivity :

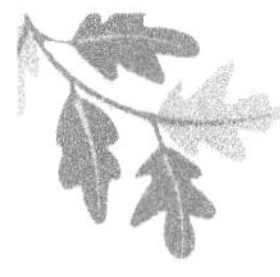

SIBO DIET
Daily Meal Planner

Date :

To Do :

M	
T	
W	
Th	
Fri	
Sat	
Sun	

Notes :

Achievement:

Meals :

Breakfast

Lunch

Dinner

Remember, you are not alone. Millions of people around the world suffer from SIBO. But by working together, we can find relief and live our best lives.

Productivity :

◯ ◯ ◯ ◯ ◯

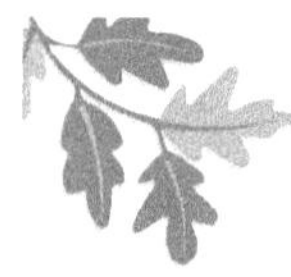

SIBO DIET
Daily Meal Planner

Date :

To Do :

M	
T	
W	
Th	
Fri	
Sat	
Sun	

Notes :

Remember, you are not alone. Millions of people around the world suffer from SIBO. But by working together, we can find relief and live our best lives.

Achievement:

Meals :

Breakfast

Lunch

Dinner

Productivity :

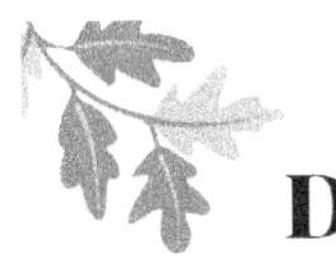

SIBO DIET
Daily Meal Planner

Date :

To Do :

M	
T	
W	
Th	
Fri	
Sat	
Sun	

Notes :

Remember, you are not alone. Millions of people around the world suffer from SIBO. But by working together, we can find relief and live our best lives.

Achievement:

Meals :

Breakfast

Lunch

Dinner

Productivity :

SIBO DIET
Daily Meal Planner

Date :

To Do :

M	
T	
W	
Th	
Fri	
Sat	
Sun	

Notes :

Remember, you are not alone. Millions of people around the world suffer from SIBO. But by working together, we can find relief and live our best lives.

Achievement:

Meals :

Breakfast

Lunch

Dinner

Productivity :

○ ○ ○ ○ ○

SIBO DIET
Daily Meal Planner

Date :

To Do :

M	
T	
W	
Th	
Fri	
Sat	
Sun	

Achievement:

Meals :

Breakfast

Lunch

Dinner

Notes :

Remember, you are not alone. Millions of people around the world suffer from SIBO. But by working together, we can find relief and live our best lives.

Productivity :

○ ○ ○ ○ ○

SIBO DIET
Daily Meal Planner

Date :

To Do :

M	
T	
W	
Th	
Fri	
Sat	
Sun	

Notes :

Remember, you are not alone. Millions of people around the world suffer from SIBO. But by working together, we can find relief and live our best lives.

Achievement:

Meals :

Breakfast

Lunch

Dinner

Productivity :

SIBO DIET
Daily Meal Planner

Date :

To Do :

M	
T	
W	
Th	
Fri	
Sat	
Sun	

Notes :

Achievement:

Meals :

Breakfast

Lunch

Dinner

Remember, you are not alone. Millions of people around the world suffer from SIBO. But by working together, we can find relief and live our best lives.

Productivity :

SIBO DIET
Daily Meal Planner

Date :

To Do :

M	
T	
W	
Th	
Fri	
Sat	
Sun	

Notes :

Remember, you are not alone. Millions of people around the world suffer from SIBO. But by working together, we can find relief and live our best lives.

Achievement:

Meals :

Breakfast

Lunch

Dinner

Productivity :

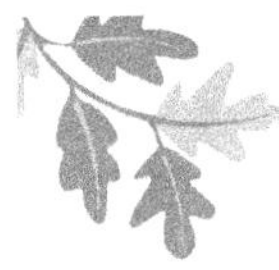

SIBO DIET
Daily Meal Planner

Date :

To Do :

M	
T	
W	
Th	
Fri	
Sat	
Sun	

Notes :

Remember, you are not alone. Millions of people around the world suffer from SIBO. But by working together, we can find relief and live our best lives.

Achievement:

Meals :

Breakfast

Lunch

Dinner

Productivity :

○ ○ ○ ○ ○

SIBO DIET
Daily Meal Planner

Date :

To Do :

M	
T	
W	
Th	
Fri	
Sat	
Sun	

Notes :

Remember, you are not alone. Millions of people around the world suffer from SIBO. But by working together, we can find relief and live our best lives.

Achievement:

Meals :

Breakfast

Lunch

Dinner

Productivity :

○ ○ ○ ○ ○

SIBO DIET
Daily Meal Planner

Date :

To Do :

M	
T	
W	
Th	
Fri	
Sat	
Sun	

Notes :

Remember, you are not alone. Millions of people around the world suffer from SIBO. But by working together, we can find relief and live our best lives.

Achievement:

Meals :

Breakfast

Lunch

Dinner

Productivity :

SIBO DIET
Daily Meal Planner

Date :

To Do :

M	
T	
W	
Th	
Fri	
Sat	
Sun	

Notes :

Achievement:

Meals :

Breakfast

Lunch

Dinner

Remember, you are not alone. Millions of people around the world suffer from SIBO. But by working together, we can find relief and live our best lives.

Productivity :

◯ ◯ ◯ ◯ ◯

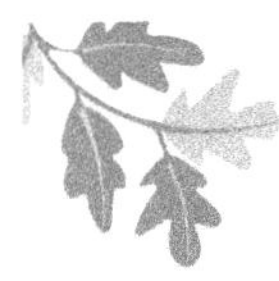

SIBO DIET
Daily Meal Planner

Date :

To Do :

M	
T	
W	
Th	
Fri	
Sat	
Sun	

Notes :

Achievement:

Meals :

Breakfast

Lunch

Dinner

Remember, you are not alone. Millions of people around the world suffer from SIBO. But by working together, we can find relief and live our best lives.

Productivity :

SIBO DIET
Daily Meal Planner

Date :

To Do :

M	
T	
W	
Th	
Fri	
Sat	
Sun	

Notes :

Remember, you are not alone. Millions of people around the world suffer from SIBO. But by working together, we can find relief and live our best lives.

Achievement:

Meals :

Breakfast

Lunch

Dinner

Productivity :

○ ○ ○ ○ ○

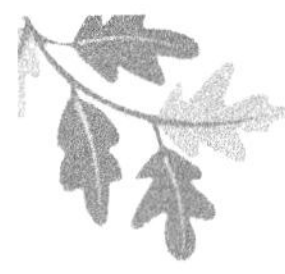

SIBO DIET
Daily Meal Planner

Date :

To Do :

M	
T	
W	
Th	
Fri	
Sat	
Sun	

Notes :

Remember, you are not alone. Millions of people around the world suffer from SIBO. But by working together, we can find relief and live our best lives.

Achievement:

Meals :

Breakfast

Lunch

Dinner

Productivity :

〇 〇 〇 〇 〇

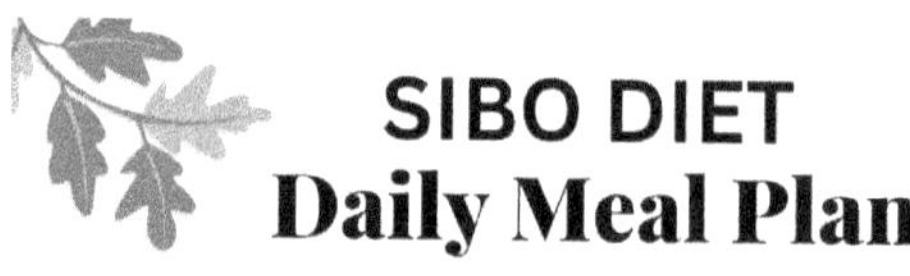

SIBO DIET
Daily Meal Planner

Date :

To Do :

M	
T	
W	
Th	
Fri	
Sat	
Sun	

Notes :

Remember, you are not alone. Millions of people around the world suffer from SIBO. But by working together, we can find relief and live our best lives.

Achievement:

Meals :

Breakfast

Lunch

Dinner

Productivity :

○ ○ ○ ○ ○

SIBO DIET
Daily Meal Planner

Date :

To Do :

M	
T	
W	
Th	
Fri	
Sat	
Sun	

Notes :

Remember, you are not alone. Millions of people around the world suffer from SIBO. But by working together, we can find relief and live our best lives.

Achievement:

Meals :

Breakfast

Lunch

Dinner

Productivity :

SIBO DIET
Daily Meal Planner

Date :

To Do :

M	
T	
W	
Th	
Fri	
Sat	
Sun	

Notes :

Remember, you are not alone. Millions of people around the world suffer from SIBO. But by working together, we can find relief and live our best lives.

Achievement:

Meals :

Breakfast

Lunch

Dinner

Productivity :

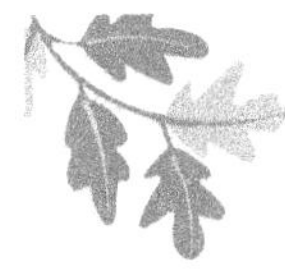

SIBO DIET
Daily Meal Planner

Date :

To Do :

M	
T	
W	
Th	
Fri	
Sat	
Sun	

Notes :

Remember, you are not alone. Millions of people around the world suffer from SIBO. But by working together, we can find relief and live our best lives.

Achievement:

Meals :

Breakfast

Lunch

Dinner

Productivity :

SIBO DIET
Daily Meal Planner

Date :

To Do :

M	
T	
W	
Th	
Fri	
Sat	
Sun	

Notes :

Remember, you are not alone. Millions of people around the world suffer from SIBO. But by working together, we can find relief and live our best lives.

Achievement:

Meals :

Breakfast

Lunch

Dinner

Productivity :

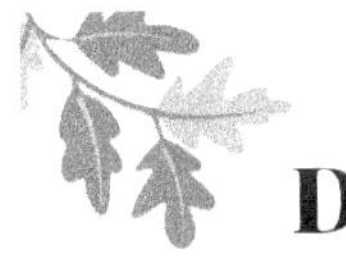

SIBO DIET
Daily Meal Planner

Date :

To Do :

M	
T	
W	
Th	
Fri	
Sat	
Sun	

Notes :

Remember, you are not alone. Millions of people around the world suffer from SIBO. But by working together, we can find relief and live our best lives.

Achievement:

Meals :

Breakfast

Lunch

Dinner

Productivity :

SIBO DIET
Daily Meal Planner

Date :

To Do :

M	
T	
W	
Th	
Fri	
Sat	
Sun	

Notes :

Remember, you are not alone. Millions of people around the world suffer from SIBO. But by working together, we can find relief and live our best lives.

Achievement:

Meals :

Breakfast

Lunch

Dinner

Productivity :

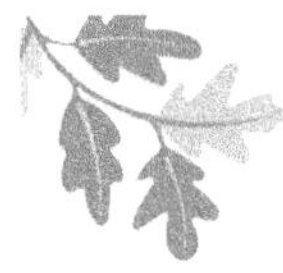

SIBO DIET
Daily Meal Planner

Date :

To Do :

M	
T	
W	
Th	
Fri	
Sat	
Sun	

Notes :

Remember, you are not alone. Millions of people around the world suffer from SIBO. But by working together, we can find relief and live our best lives.

Achievement:

Meals :

Breakfast

Lunch

Dinner

Productivity :

SIBO DIET
Daily Meal Planner

Date :

To Do :

M	
T	
W	
Th	
Fri	
Sat	
Sun	

Notes :

Remember, you are not alone. Millions of people around the world suffer from SIBO. But by working together, we can find relief and live our best lives.

Achievement:

Meals :

Breakfast

Lunch

Dinner

Productivity :

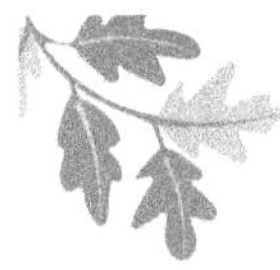

SIBO DIET
Daily Meal Planner

Date :

To Do :

M	
T	
W	
Th	
Fri	
Sat	
Sun	

Notes :

Remember, you are not alone. Millions of people around the world suffer from SIBO. But by working together, we can find relief and live our best lives.

Achievement:

Meals :

Breakfast

Lunch

Dinner

Productivity :